The Magic of Asafetida

For Cooking and Healing

Dueep Jyot Singh

Natural Remedy Series

Mendon Cottage Books

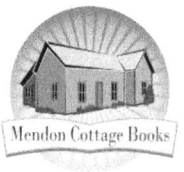

JD-Biz Publishing

Download Free Books!

http://MendonCottageBooks.com

Our books are available at

1. Amazon.com

2. Barnes and Noble

3. Itunes

4. Kobo

5. Smashwords

6. Google Play Books

Table of Contents

Introduction

This book introduces you to one of the most notorious of all spices – the Asafetida. Many people do not use it, as a flavoring ingredient in their foods, because they say it smells. Nevertheless, this spice has been an integral part of the cuisine found near the regions, of the NWFP , which is now called Afghanistan.

My father was born in this area, and he talks about remembering Pakhtoons crossing the border with their backpacks full of dried fruit, Asafetida, and spices, which they used to grow on the mountains of Afghanistan. This Asafetida was collected as sap from the taproot of an indigenous plant, which grew extensively all over that region.

He remembers, running after the gruff Afghani salesmen saying "Khan-a, Kharo Moshai" which was a greeting to the Khan. In return, a gruff baritone would always answer Khara Moshay in return. These vendors sold their products, from door to door, and one knew that they were going to be getting original spices, dry fruits, as well as natural Asafetida without any sort of adulteration. That is why this spice is so expensive.

The call of these door to door salesman always used to be "Heeng-o-jeera" which meant Asafetida and cumin seeds. That is why, Asafetida cannot do without cumin seeds and vice versa, when you are cooking a traditionally Eastern dish.

It is on par with saffron, which is often adulterated with other dried flower stamens. Pure Asafetida powder is going to have its particular smell and that is why it is not used more than one pinch to give any dish, a taste of onions or leeks.

Since ancient times, Asafetida has been used as a medicine to cure lots of ailments. In the West, it was considered to be the devils dung, because of its fetid odor and lumpy yellowish dung like look. That is why it was used in black magic rituals. No wonder it got a notorious reputation in medieval times.

Any woman buying this spice would immediately be labeled as a Devil's disciple, and would either be burned at the stake or ducked in the nearest pond. However, this sort of ritualism was definitely not a part of Eastern cuisine, or Eastern ancient medical alternative medicine tradition.

This is also known as giant fennel, and as fennel is traditionally called ajowain, Asafetida was called jowani badian- the badian meaning excellent in the vernacular. So *excellent fennel*!

Tempering in the Indian subcontinent cannot do without Asafetida. Every proud housewife has this ingredient in her kitchen, and all she has to do is put clarified butter in the wok, a hefty pinch of Asafetida, and some onion seeds and mustard seeds. When they start spluttering, she empties out her lentils dish or meat dish on top of this red-hot tempering oil. It will be served sizzling hot to people who enjoy their food.

In many parts of India, many people do not eat onions and garlic, because traditionally, they consider these herbs of not being a part of their ancient and traditional religious beliefs. That is why a pinch of Asafetida was enough to give the food an "onion taste."

South Indian food, traditionally the sambhar you eat with traditional vegetarian foods like idli and dosai are tempered with a small bit of Asafetida, so that this food is acceptable to even all those people who are extremely particular about garlic, and onions in their diets! This tempering is called Popu in South India and Tadka in North India. That is where you are going to add a touch of cumin seeds also to add more zest to the curry or to the nonvegetarian dish like lentils.

Asafetida has normally such a strong odor, that it is kept far away from other spices. Otherwise the other spices are going to capture that supposedly fetid smell of raw Asafetida.

Like I told you earlier, this natural resin is adulterated by people mixing a small quantity of Asafetida with very finely ground wheat bran and wheat flour.

If you buy it from an original dealer, he is going to give it to you with just this tiny hole at the bottom of the container which is going to serve as the sprinkler to pepper your cuisine. But I would suggest that you heat it in clarified butter, so that the flavor gets milder and more appealing.

How to Grow Asafetida

Growing Asafetida in your garden? Whoever could think of that? But really speaking, this plant is rather appealing, because it belongs to the ferula family with very attractive foliage. Even though this is a perennial plant, it is going to bloom only once in its lifetime, and then it is going to die. That is why farmers make sure that this plant is used to the utmost before blooming, so that they can take full advantage of the sap from its stem and from its roots.

Even though this plant is native to Afghanistan, did you know that Asafetida is being grown extensively in desert areas in the US? That is because it does not bother much about water. So if your area is dry, with plenty of sun, make sure to have a little bit of Asafetida growing in your garden, just for fun.

This plant can grow up to 1 m in height and it can spread to another 1 m sideways. So make sure that your plant has plenty of elbow space to elbow out the competition.

The scientific name of this plant is Ferula assafoetida. It is a hardy herb and perennial.

Harvesting the Sap

Shallow cuts are made in the plant's stem and also in its roots, and the sap collected. This gum is whitish – grayish in color, when it is collected fresh, but on exposure to the atmosphere and to the sun, it grows into an amber – golden color.

The roots of this plant are massive, and pulpy. That is why more people extract Asafetida from the roots than from the stems which are hollow and thick with plant tissue which contains this gum.

64% of Asafetida is going to be made about resin and the rest is made up of volatile oil, gum and ash. The Persian word aza or resin along with the Latin word fetidus made up this word in English. In the Indian subcontinent, it is called Hing, ingu, inguva or such etymologically similar names.

Of course in the West, apart from being called Devil's dung, you can also hear it being called merde du diable, Teufelsdreck and so on.

Type of Soil?

This plant can grow in any type of soil, basic, neutral and acidic, loamy, sandy and clay. So you do not have to bother much about the pH level.

You must choose soil that is well drained. Almost all types of soil work; sandy, loam or clay work well for asafetida. It is a herbaceous perennial and tends to tolerate acidic, neutral and basic soil pH levels. The soil does need to be well-drained, so stay away from clay soil.

Asafetida loves the sun, so no wonder the ancient Greeks knew all about a herb similar to it, growing in the sunny lands of Cyrene. But that herb died out around Alexander the Great's Time.

So, no shade for this plant and allow 6 feet distance between growing plants.

Watering Your Plant

Do not over water. As this is basically a plant which is native to dry areas without too much access to water, the soil has to be completely dry before you decide to moisturize it again. That is going to take anywhere between 3 to 4 days. Standing water or waterlogged Asafetida beds are going to have visiting plants, which are definitely not what you want.

In fact, this is an excellent plant, to grow in areas subject to draught. A little bit of moisture is going to do very well for it. That is why many people have been growing this plant since ancient times in the deserts of North Africa.

This plant needs to be kept warm in the winter, especially if you are in a three – eight climate zone. Just apply some mulch made of bracken in a 2 inches thick layer on the seedlings or small plants, if you want.

Sowing the Seedlings

I would suggest you begin the seedlings by sowing the seeds in 6 to 12 inches deep pots. The seedlings can be found at nurseries especially during the autumn season when it is the best time to plant the seeds, and then transplant the seedlings to their permanent homes. By this time, it is winter, so cover the small plants with a layer of bracken mulch.

Remember to transplant it only once. That is because the Roots, which are fleshy and really long do not enjoy too much of movement, once they have fixed themselves in some particular area.

In the Indian subcontinent, any sort of pests, and attacking this plant is going to be treated with a natural pesticide made up of neem oil. Empty out 250 g of neem oil in 5 L of water and spray your plants with this natural and healthy pesticide.

Asafetida to Heal

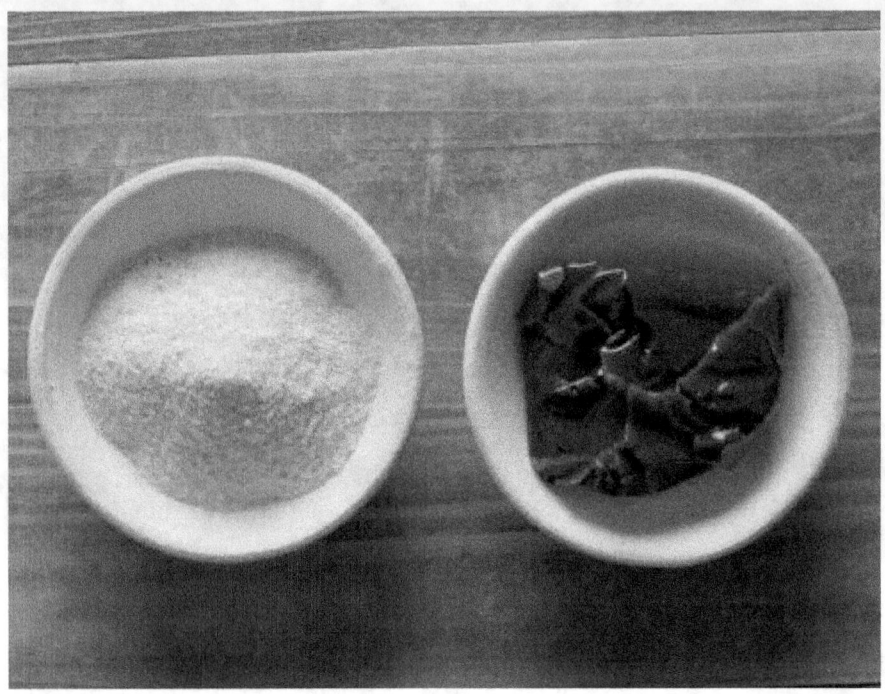

Since ancient times, Asafetida has been an important part of alternative medicine, because traditionally, this is the easiest way in which one can get rid of constipation as well as flatulence. All the digestive tasty and spicy "bullets/balls" made locally in the Indian subcontinent, is going to have Asafetida in it.

People in Thailand, suffering from tummy aches, brought about by constipation, indigestion, or other digestion related problems are going to have a mixture of three pinches of Asafetida in a cup of water, boiled down into a tincture – until the water is half the quantity – and then rub it all over the affected area. You can consider this to be quite a good massage which gets your digestive system up and running again.

Believe it or not, in ancient medicine, this Asafetida was considered to be an antiseptic, anti-flatulent, blood purifier, painkiller, germicidal, digestive and an anti-phlegmatic herbal cure it all. It is painkilling properties can be used in massage oils, as well as in curing aching feet, where you are going to apply a paste of a pinch of Asafetida, in just this little bit of water to that aching tooth.

This is the best application for pain relief.

Historical fact talks about a Canadian officer, who was injured in the abdomen, during a hunting accident, and was put under the care of an American Army doctor and surgeon, William Beaumont. Even though the wounds were healed properly, the area was open, because of a fistula, which could not be closed with catgut. Dr. Beaumont took this as an excellent opportunity to try different experiments, and that is why he did plenty of pioneering studies in the digestive process and the gastric process.

He made up a mixture of around 30 drops of Asafetida tincture, mixed with some muriatic acid, and wine and applied it directly into the fistula. He applied this combination without fail, three times a day, and found to his great joy, that the infection had been cured. So alright, Asafetida did the healing, but it was the alcohol in the wind, which prevented future infection.

So a little bit of experimenting with spices and herbs came into use to save the life of a gallant Canadian officer in the 19th century. In the same manner, when fatality rates during the first world war began to grow into epidemic proportions, the doctors decided to make up a series of medicines, based on Asafetida. However, all the research done by them, at that time and all the positive results have somehow been overlooked by modern researchers in the 21st century.

Let me tell you something amusing about Asafetida – in many parts of Afghanistan, especially in the area called Pakhtoonwa and even in Kashmir, India, anybody suffering from infectious diseases is immediately told to tie up a cotton bag full of Asafetida, on the arm or around the neck.

To me it does almost the same duty as the Western Orange pomander, which was used in medieval times supposedly to ward off fever and infection. The same thing is being done in the East with an Asafetida pomander! Nevertheless, you can also consider this to be a warning signal – I smell *something* around you. Does your mama know that you are out, you infectious little specimen you?

Fishing Bait

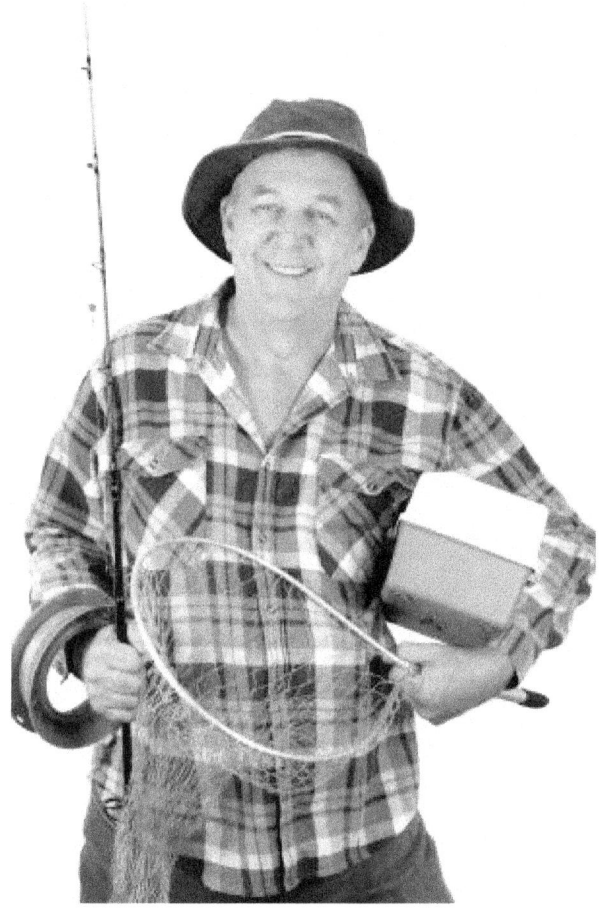

Try fishing the next time with asafetida bait!

Now this is something which is going to be very interesting to all those people who intend to spend the weekend fishing for pike, and catfish. Just try making small balls of dough, in which a little bit of Asafetida has been added. I do not know whether this works on someone to, but in the 1930s, every serious fisherman had this particular natural fish bait added to his fishing basket.

Ceremonial Magic

In medieval times, this was called the Devil's dung, in England, and other countries around it. But they were not the only ones who considered Asafetida to have anything to do with spirits. A traditional Jamaican witch doctor always added a little bit of Asafetida, in rituals, so that the bad spirits kept away. Also, good spirits were not affected with Asafetida, so this was both a repellent as well as the protective medium.

Even ancient ceremonial magic going back to King Solomon's times spoke about Asafetida as one of the ingredients which would not only protect the enchanter, when he was conjuring up demons, but this would bind the demons to him.

In Alexander's time there was a plant belonging to the same fennel family called Silphium. This was obtained only in North Africa in a place named Cyrene. This was like Asafetida but was considerably milder in taste, as well as in smell. However, the plant soon died out, and so Asafetida brought directly from Persia, by Alexander's soldiers coming back to Greece, began to make this plant more well known.

 Cooks as well as doctors began to look at the different ways in which they could utilize this plant to its maximum benefit.

In ancient Eastern as well as Jewish literature, it is always said that one should not eat too much of Asafetida, as well as mustard in the summer, along with spicy food.

Throat Infections

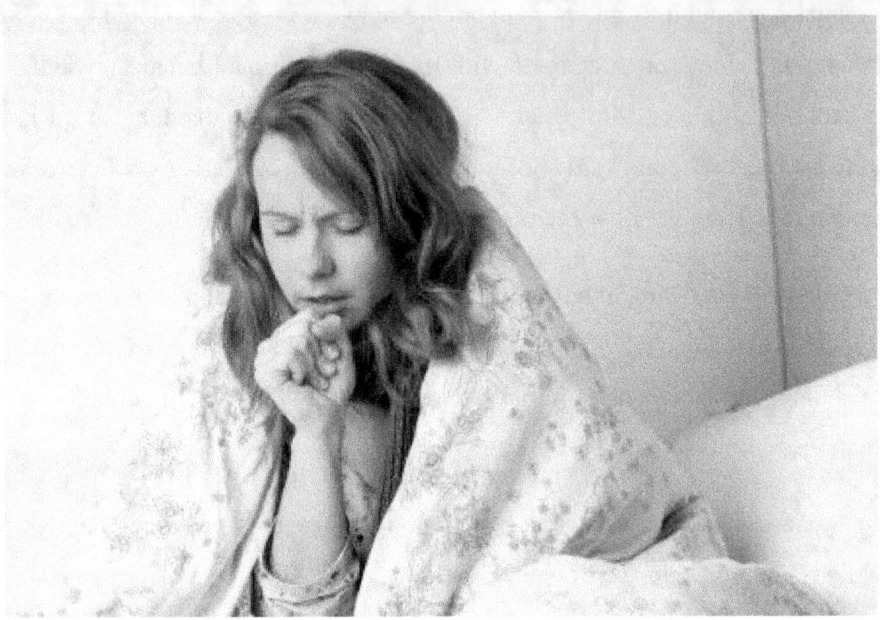

Even up to the 20s and the 30s, Edwardian and Victorian mothers in the United States and in Europe thought that their kids could get cured of throat infections by wrapping a piece of cloth with Asafetida in it around the neck. I do not think that an external application of this herb is going to help.

Instead, the mothers could have got an infection free kid by making him gargle with hot water in which a little Asafetida had been dissolved.

In the same way, if they suffered from phlegm due to a cough or cold, all they had to do was chop up pieces of fresh ginger, sprinkle some heeng on the ginger and make the kids suck this. This would clear up the infection as

---

well as make sure that there was no possibility of potential future infection, thanks to the ginger and Asafetida.

Influenza Remedy

If you are suffering from influenza, try drinking water boiled with 3 g each of cinnamon, cumin seeds, and a pinch of Asafetida thrice a day, for 3 to 4 days until you are cured completely.

Urinary Infections

Urinary infections can be cured by roasting a little bit of Asafetida on the griddle, and dissolving it in water. Drink this liquid twice a day until you are cured completely.

Bronchitis Cure

Now this is a timeworn remedy, which you may want to use to cure people suffering from bronchitis. Add a pinch of Asafetida to a glassful of hot water, in which you have put in three raisins. Boil this once and then cool. Make the patient drink this two times a day. This combination is good for healing. Bronchitis, as well as taking care of any sort of possible future throat irritations in the bronchial region.

Here is one tasty, delicious, spicy digestive mix which is going to make certain that you never are troubled with stomach as well as digestion problems.

Heeng Spicy Mix

This digestive mix is normally sold by enterprising urchins in the Indian subcontinent, anywhere near a place on the roadside where plenty of street food is being sold. That is because they know that most of their clients are going to overreach their digestive capacities, and find themselves too stuffed for words after an eat-athon. That is when the budding businessman slowly sidles up and says suavely, "sir ji will be wanting special hing churan no? Just be taking one big pinch after eating and no problems in Tummy. Just be putting it in hot water and drinking."

So you buy it. You eat it. It is so tasty. You take one spoonful, instead of a pinch – 2 g, thinking the more the merrier. And before you know it you have finished the container of 20 spoonfuls.

And you come down with a greater tummy ache. Been there, done that.

This is what the mixture is going to consist of –

3 tablespoons each of cumin seeds, black pepper, rock salt, white pepper, and Royal cumin, 1 tablespoon aniseed, 2 tablespoon dried ginger and 1/8 teaspoon full of Asafetida. All of these are roasted with a little bit of sodium bicarbonate.

You can either take this in powdered form, in water or roasted – remember, not more than one pinch, because I have added all the spices in large proportions. 1/8 teaspoon of Asafetida is definitely going to be detrimental to your digestive system and to your future healthy state.

This is also an amazing way in which you can prevent bad breath. That is because your digestive system is working perfectly. So there is no chance of bad breath ever occurring. Elementary, my dear Watson.

Arthritis Oil

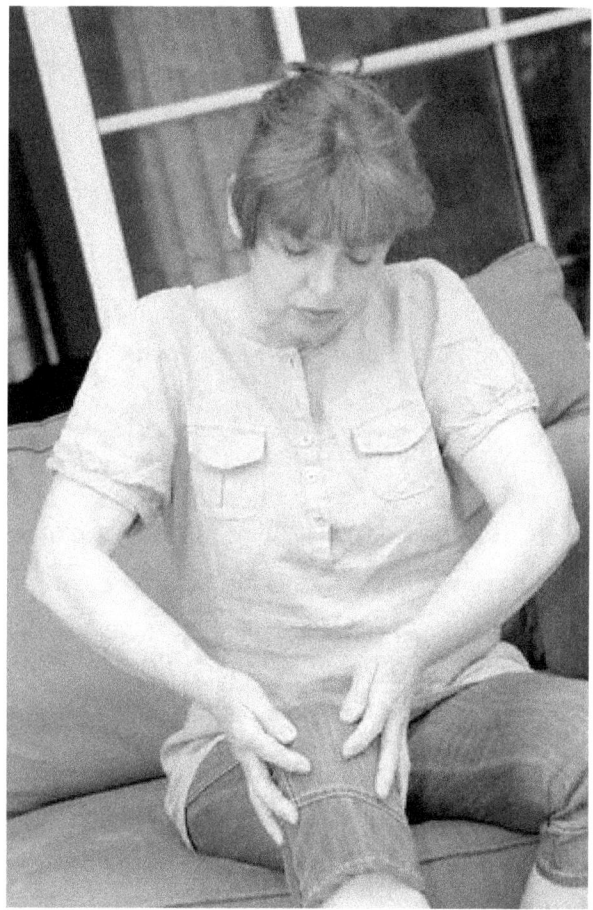

This is a traditional arthritis cure and remedy, which is excellent for painful joints. You normally use this as massaging oil in winter. This one is definitely not for those with sensitive nostrils. That is because it is going to have two cloves of garlic, 1 tablespoon of rock salt, and two pinches of Asafetida in mustard oil. Three of these ingredients are rather smelly. Bring the oil to a boil and then allow to cool and strain. Cover-up with a cloth after the massage has been done for about 10 min..

You may also want to add half a teaspoon of this arthritis oil in a cup of hot milk, before you go to bed. Not only is the hot milk going to give you a good night's sleep, but you are also going to find you not suffering from any joint pain during the night.

Strengthening a Heart

We are not talking about brave hearts here, and courage, but possibly this has to be a character aspect of those persons suffering from weak hearts genetically or due to some ailments.

Make up a mixture of these very powerful and healing ingredients – you are going to take only three pinches of this mixed with rock salt 3 to 4 times a day. This is supposed to cure heart problems, and strengthen the muscles of your heart.

Healthy Heart Mix

Grind together 12 seed – less raisins, and 12 seeded dates. To this add 5 g of Asafetida. 1 teaspoon is 6 g.

1 1/2 teaspoons of powdered green cardamom and cinnamon with two pinches of rock salt is added to this mixture.

This powerful mixture has to be put in an airtight glass bottle. Take a pinch, after every four hours. This is going to give your heart a boost, as well as add to the rejuvenating and invigorating effect on your muscular tissues.

A pinch of Roasted Asafetida taken with warm water is considered to be a really good warming drink, especially in the winter when you want to feel energetic. It also energizes your body's circulatory system and purifies your blood.

Suffering from Diarrhea/Dysentery

This is going to happen, when you have been eating lots of things, without bothering about their fresh or stale state, or you have been overeating. Food eaten in unhygienic conditions and contaminated food can also cause diarrhea and dysentery.

Mango Cure

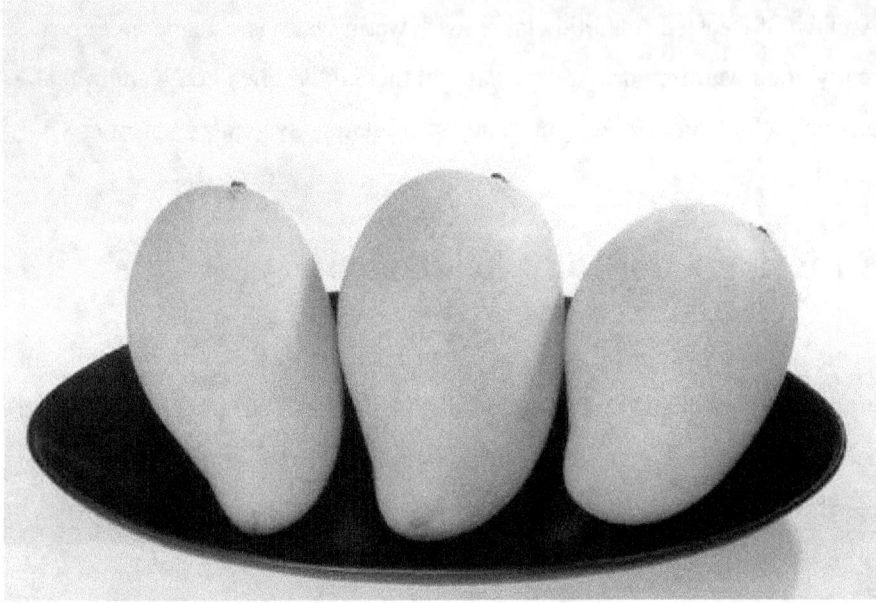

This is a rather ancient and time-tested remedy, and it was very much in use in the summers, because that was the time mangoes were in season. So many children got really ill, because they had been eating raw fruit in the summer, including raw mangoes. That is the reason why mothers made sure that they had the seed of one Mango always there in the kitchen.

The seed was roasted on the hot dry griddle and the outer covering cracked open so that you could get to the soft part inside the seed. Then roast two pinches of Asafetida. Mix it with the soft parts and grind. Add two pinches of rock salt so that the child does not suffer from dehydration. Give the patient teaspoonful of this powder twice a day with buttermilk. This is going to cure diarrhea.

If you do not have buttermilk around, you could roast Asafetida, as well as cumin seeds separately. Then powder them together and roast with 2 tablespoons full of clarified butter.

Grind these together when you have cooled down, the spice and Herb mixture. Take half a teaspoon with warm water twice a day, to cure any sort of chronic dysentery.

So How Do You Make Buttermilk?

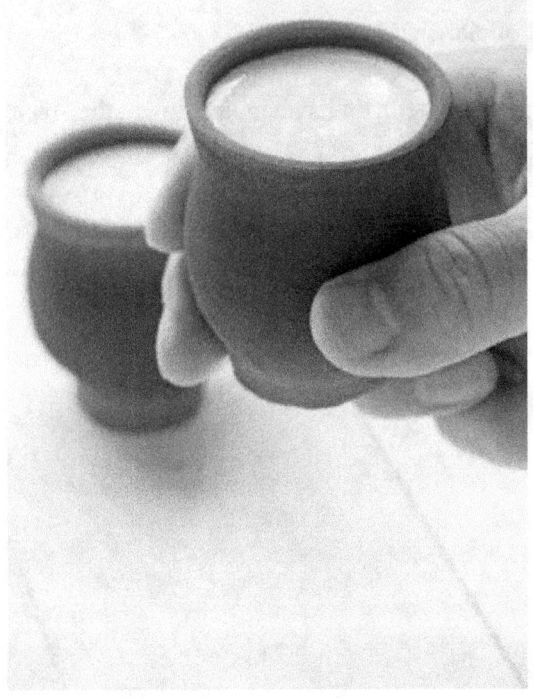

Lassi not served in traditional clay pots? Half the fun is lost.

Traditional buttermilk is definitely not for weight watchers. Julia Child would have loved this rich and healthy dish, because it had plenty of butter in it.

To make traditional buttermilk you need **one cup of full fat, full cream curd.** Buffaloes milk available in Thailand, Indonesia, Malaysia and other Oriental countries as well as in the Indian subcontinent is preferred to make this yogurt , because the people living in these countries do not mind a bit of obesity, especially when they are confronted with health giving milk products.

To this, add 6 to 8 mint leaves. Salt-and-pepper to taste along with half a cup of water.

All of these are gathered together in one blender and allowed to blend for about 30 seconds. This is then poured into tall glasses, along with half a teaspoonful of ground and roasted cumin seeds and just this little touch of Asafetida roasted with the cumin.

Making Clarified Butter the Traditional Way

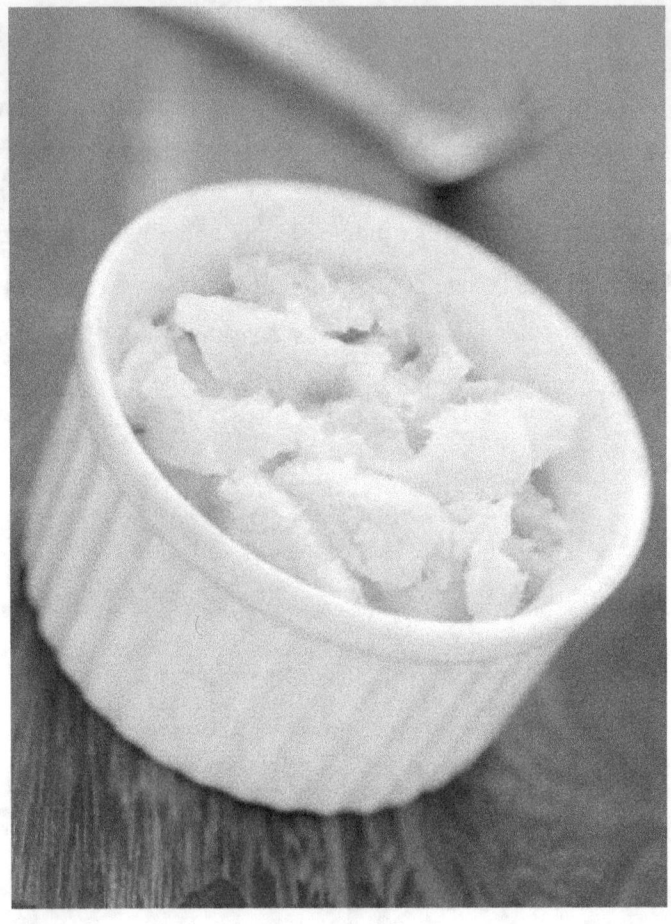

This has solidified. So I think that it has been adulterated with vegetable oils. Traditional butter is normally grainier, more liquid and more golden amber in color.

In the same way, I am teaching you how to make clarified butter. This is the traditional method, where you are going to be selecting full cream yogurt to turn into butter. You do that by putting this yogurt along with a couple of cups of water into your blender and allowed to blend until the milky solid rises up to the surface and you are left with whey – the liquid part – and solid butter.

Put this butter on the fire, stirring constantly, so that all the milk content is cooked and removed. This content is going to be Amber – Golden in color and you need to remove it from the liquid butter, which is now getting clarified and turning into your clarified butter.

This butter is extremely concentrated. That is why you use it in just small quantities for natural remedies, or for cooking purposes.

Filter this and place this in a glass jar. Keep in a cool and dry corner of your kitchen, far away from the heat and let it gather strength and aroma. Then use your teaspoonful of cooking or tempering your food. Use within three months

Tempering Your Food with Asafetida.

Chicken in the Wok

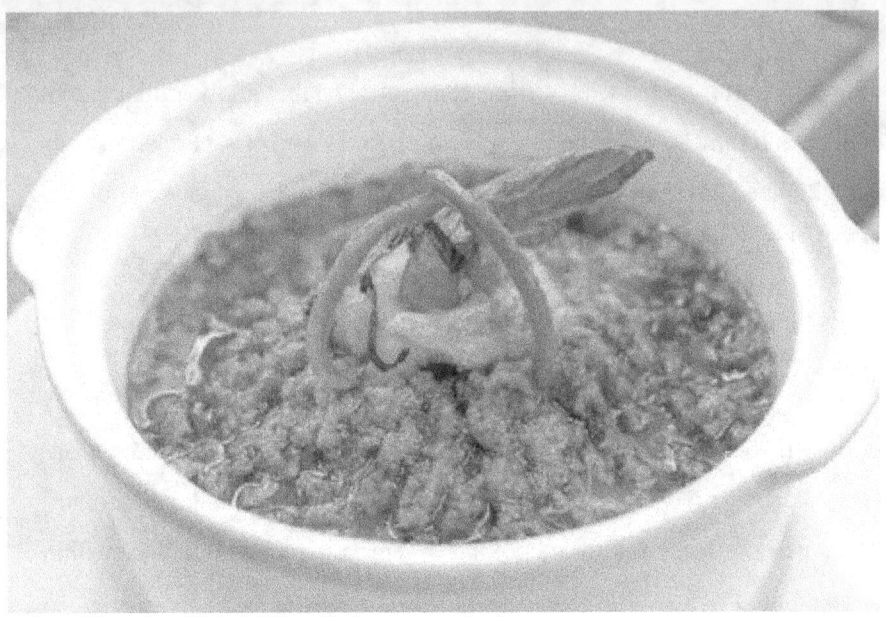

Tempered with asafoetida!

Now this is a semidry preparation of chicken, which is rich, flavorful, and to be savored by only those gourmets, who do not mind eating and Eastern dish flavored with coriander, Asafetida and fenugreek.

4 – 6 hungry people are going to enjoy this rich and spicy dish.

For that you need one medium-size chicken, or 500 g of unless chicken pieces of 3/4 inches, 6 tablespoons of clarified butter, 1 tablespoon full of coriander seeds, half a teaspoonful of fenugreek seeds, and 1 tablespoon full of green fenugreek leaves.

This original recipe calls for some special fenugreek leaves, which are found only in Kashmir. They are called kasuri methi. As I do not have them growing in my garden, I use ordinary fenugreek leaves.

Three whole red chilies. I told you it would be spicy. You can either put them whole into the dish, or slice them. If you slice them, you are going to have red-hot chicken. If you seed them you are going to have a milder chicken.

2 1/2 cloves , crushed and chopped garlic

Half a cup of tomato purée.

Six red chopped tomatoes.

Half a piece of ginger, chopped, green chilies cut into long slices. 1/4 cup of cream along with the 1/4 cup of water.

The spices are going to be one teaspoon red chili powder, two teaspoonful of ground coriander powder, 2 teaspoons salt to taste, half a cup of chopped green coriander, and one green capsicum chopped.

One tomato for garnishing. You may also add any other spices you like, like cumin seed, cinnamon turmeric, and of course a pinch of Asafetida.

Put the coriander seeds on to roast on the griddle pan.

Roast them lightly until they begin to change color, and before they turn brown instead of their original yellowish amber color, remove from heat.

Crush the coriander seeds or grind them with a rolling pin to get a coarsely powdered mix.

Heat the clarified butter in a Wok. Now, this is the wok, in which you are going to be cooking as well as serving this red-hot dish after it has been tempered with cumin seeds and Asafetida at the end of the cooking session.

Add the fenugreek seeds, and the whole red chilies and stir on low heat until the fenugreek seeds turn a little brown. Why is the kitchen not smelling of roasted chilies. That is because they are still whole and I am roasting them on low heat.

But it is better not to take any chances, because you never know with chilies. Add the onions and cook on medium heat under the onions are semitransparent. The addition is going to reduce the power of the chilies, which are also frying away merrily.

Now add the pieces of chicken and fry on a high flame, on the wok, for five, six min. We are going to do traditional stir frying and that is why we are using this wok. Stir this well so that the chicken is fried and is a nice rich golden brown color.

Add the chopped tomatoes and cook for another 5 min. on highly stirring constantly.

Add the salt, and spices, and lower the heat. Cover and cook for 10 to 15 min. in its own juice.

Add the tomato purée and chopped green coriander. Allow to cook for 2 min. on medium heat. Add the tomato, capsicum, ginger pieces and slices of green chili. Mix well.

Now, reduce the heat and add the cream. Mix well. Now is the time to add water so that you get a semidry masala. Cook for 2 min. and remove from the fire.

Now, in the tempering wok, before serving you are going to temper this with one teaspoonful of clarified butter in which you have added half a teaspoonful of cumin seeds and two pinches of Asafetida, along with some mustard seeds.

Clarified butter does not burn, so you have to guesstimate the time when you put in the meat. That is when the seeds start smoking. I am definitely not advising you to put in red chilies, though that is done in the traditional tempering of meat, because then you are going to have the neighbors calling the pesticide department to get rid of you.

Now, turn off the fire and very carefully empty the masala meat right into the smoking hot butter – spice mix. Allow the oil to sizzle one second and mix thoroughly. Serve piping hot with rice or bread – roti – or even tacos.

Conclusion

So now that you know a little more about Asafetida, ensure that you are going to be using it occasionally to keep you healthy. Also, try this out as a flavor enhancer. Do you know that a very popular cheese somewhere in France is being flavored with Asafetida? That is because roasted Asafetida gives the mild leek flavor to the cheese, which could not be obtained by adding fresh and chopped leeks and onions to it.

Remember Asafetida cannot do without cumin seeds. So next time you want to temper a dish with chilies, and spices, try this mixture of Asafetida, mustard seeds, cumin seeds, onion seeds and your already cooked vegetable lentils or meat masterpiece.

Remember that this is excellent for your digestive system so you just need a bit of it to add flavor to your food, and pep to your digestion.

If you are suffering from flatulence, take half a spoonful of lemon juice and ginger juice, along with a little bit of roasted asafetida and rock salt in cold water.

Also, if you are suffering from some tummy problems caused due to trapped. "Wind" – and this can be very distressing – try this remedy right now. Boil too big pinches of asafetida in 250 mL water until it has been reduced to half the quantity. Give it to the patient, while it is still hot. This clears up your system and also gives you relief, from discomfort and pain.

These are just some of the uses to which this versatile herb has been put down the centuries. In fact, in the East, when anyone went into hysterics, they were not given Sal volatile or made to smell a leather shoe. They were just given a sniff of asafetida to dispel all the spirits causing such a bad behavior in a spoilt human being who wanted his or her own way.

Live long and prosper with natural herbal remedies!

Author Bio

Dueep Jyot Singh is a Management and IT Professional who managed to gather Postgraduate qualifications in Management and English and Degrees in Science, French and Education while pursuing different enjoyable career options like being an hospital administrator, IT,SEO and HRD Database Manager/ trainer, movie scriptwriter, theatre artiste and public speaker, lecturer in French, Marketing and Advertising, ex-Editor of Hearts On Fire (now known as Solstice) Books Missouri USA, advice columnist and cartoonist, publisher and Aviation School trainer, ex- moderator on Medico.in, banker, student councilor ,travelogue writer … among other things! One fine morning, she decided that she had enough of killing herself by Degrees and went back to her first love -- writing. It's more enjoyable! She already has 48 published academic and 14 fiction- in- different- genre books under her belt.

When she is not designing websites or making Graphic design illustrations for clients , she is browsing through old bookshops hunting for treasures, of which she has an enviable collection – including R.L. Stevenson, O.Henry, Dornford Yates, Maurice Walsh, C.N.Williamson, Sapper, Bartimeus and the crown of her collection- Dickens "The Old Curiosity Shop," and so on… Just call her "Renaissance Woman" - collecting herbal remedies, acting like Universal Helping Hand/Agony Aunt, or escaping to her dear mountains for a bit of exploring, collecting herbs and plants, and trekking.

Check out some of the other JD-Biz Publishing books

Health Learning Series

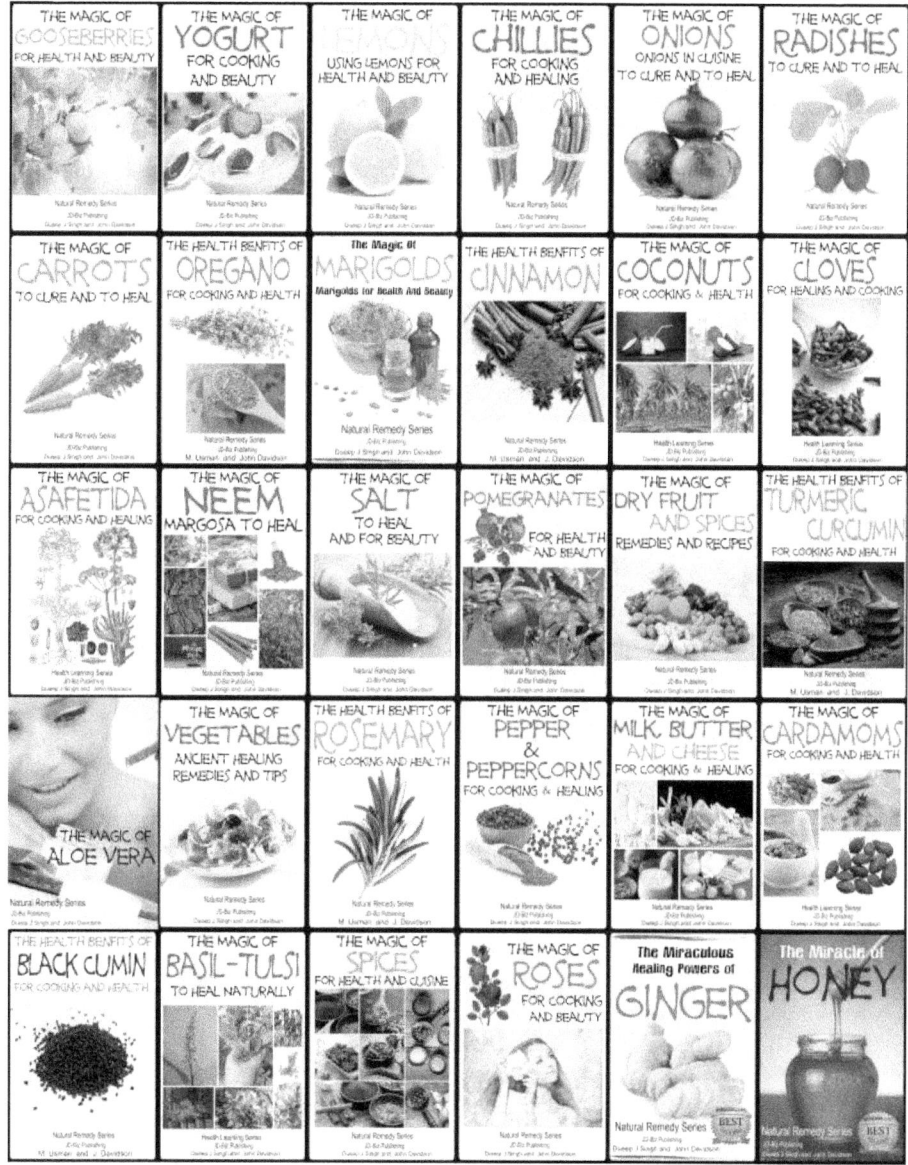

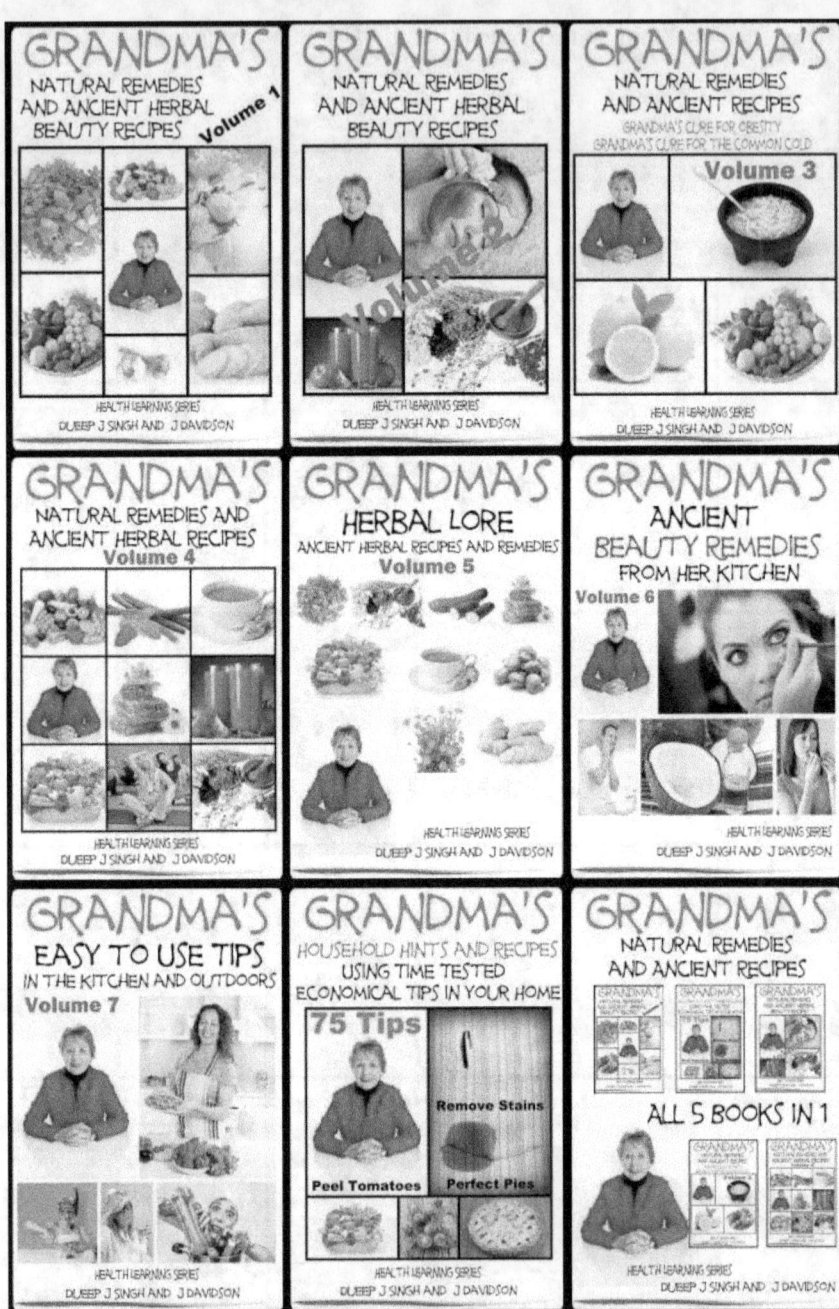

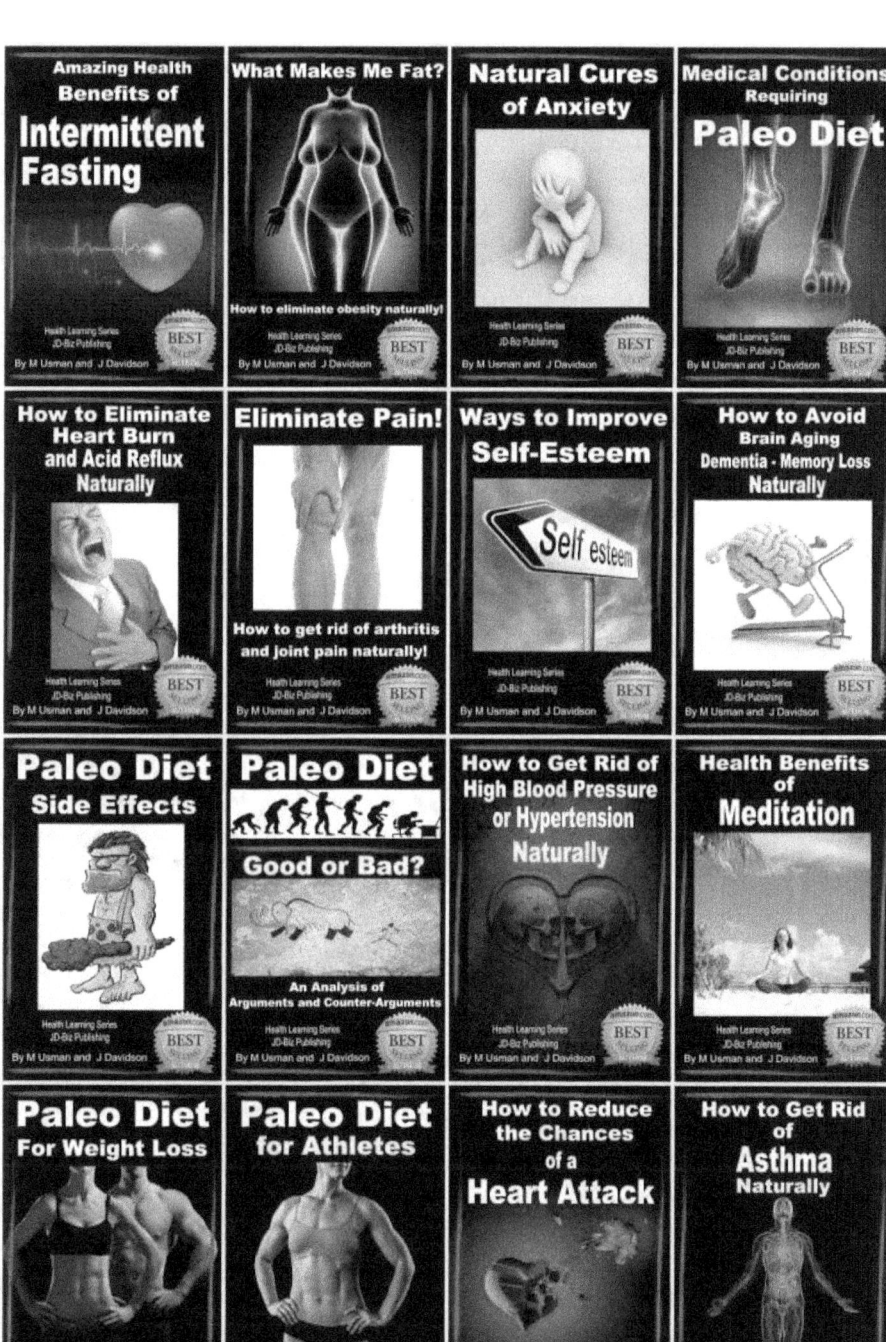

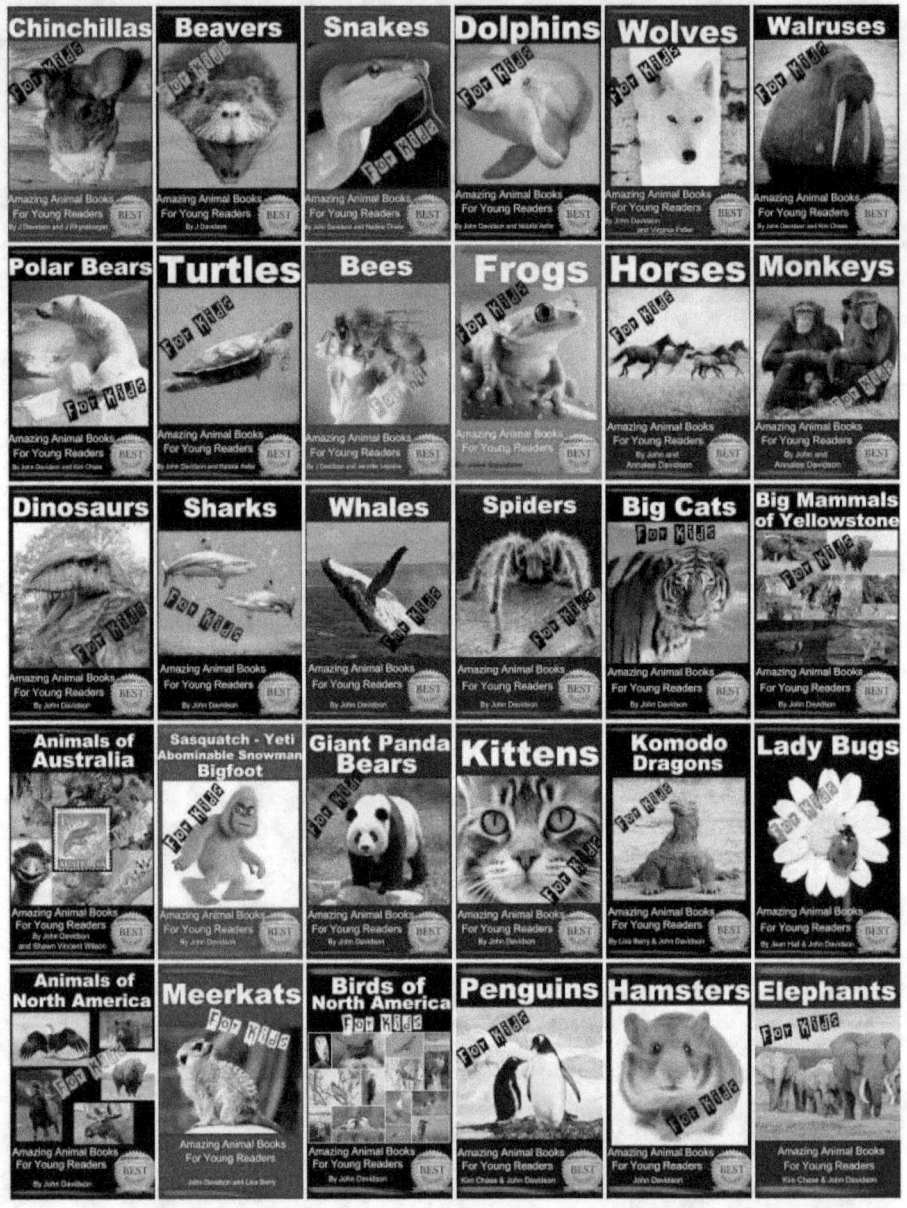

Learn To Draw Series

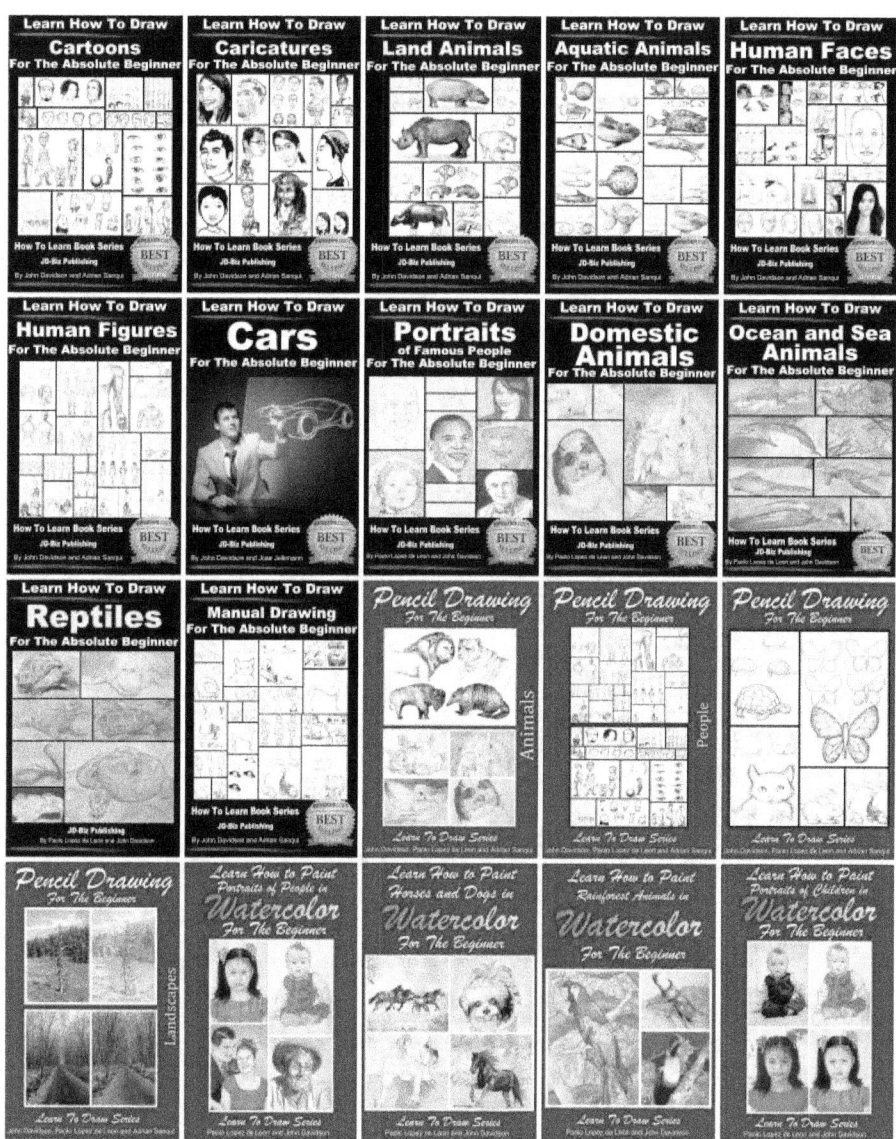

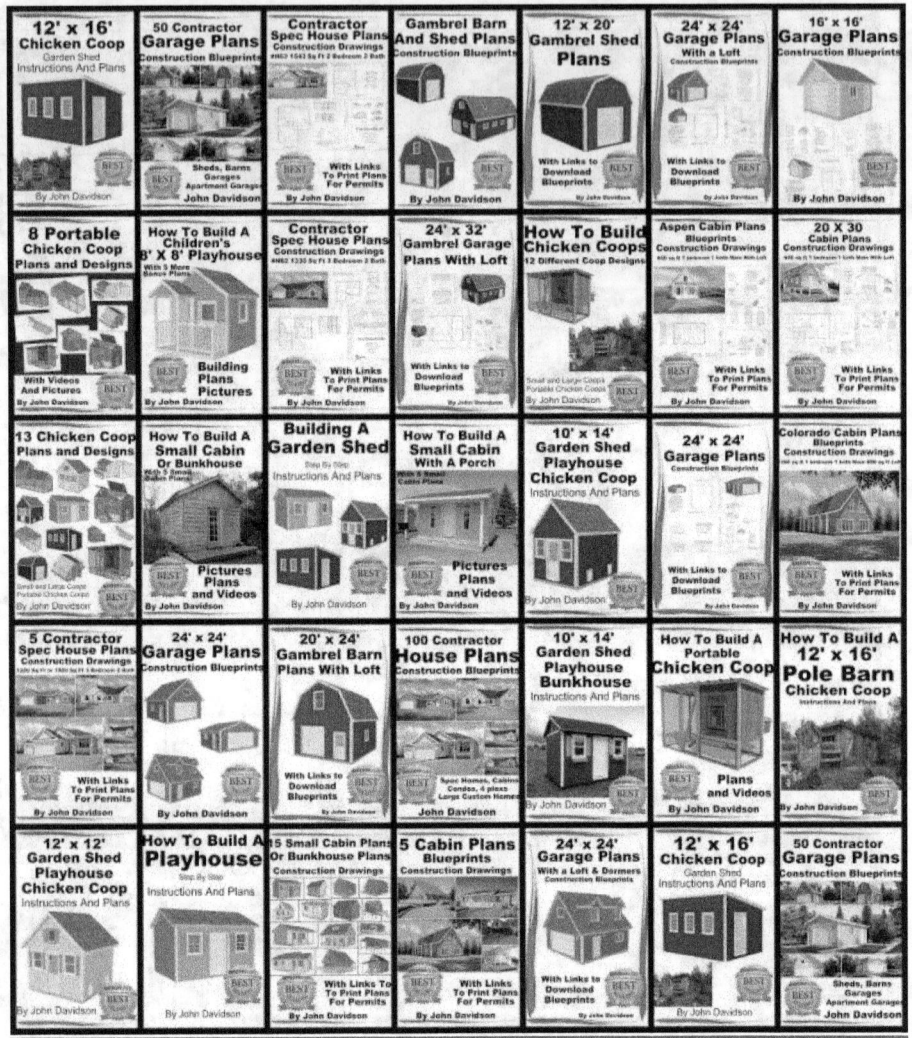

Entrepreneur Book Series

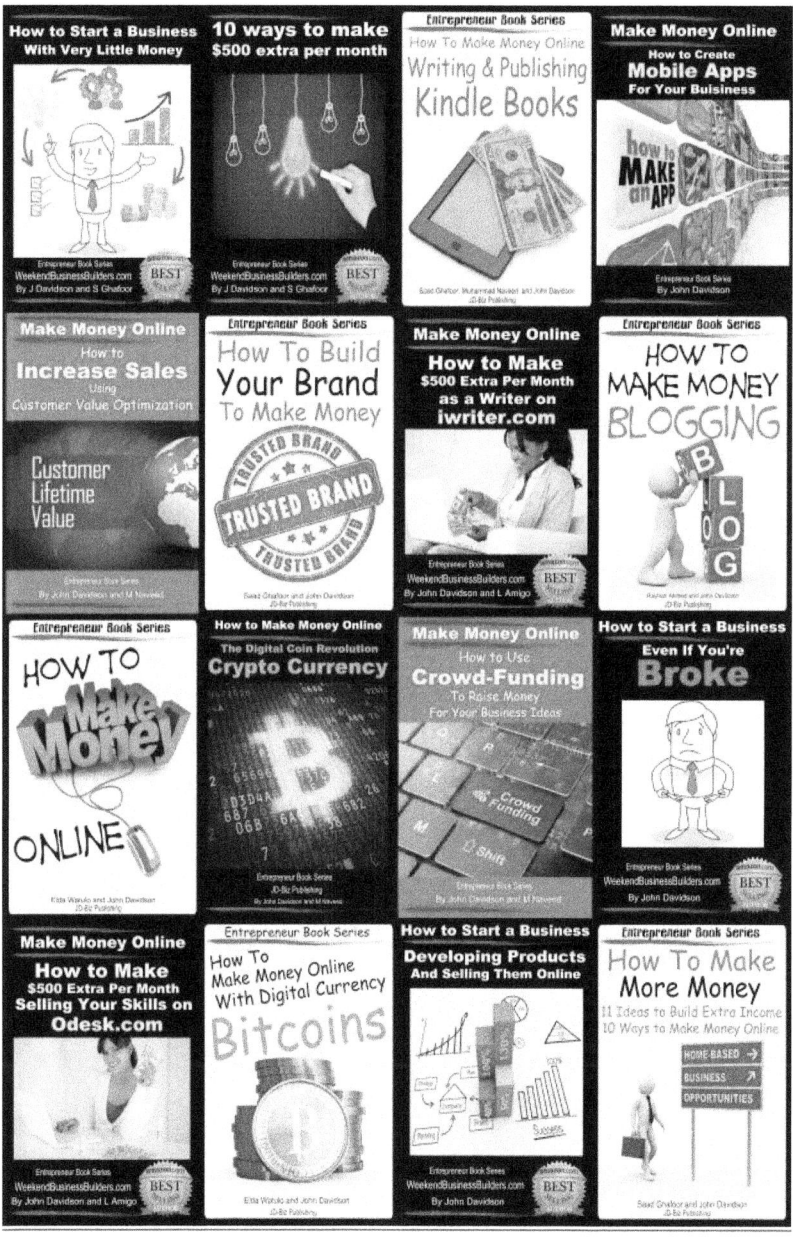

Our books are available at

1. Amazon.com

2. Barnes and Noble

3. Itunes

4. Kobo

5. Smashwords

6. Google Play Books

Download Free Books!

http://MendonCottageBooks.com

Publisher

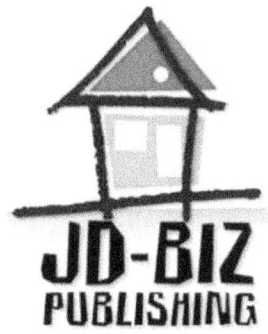

JD-Biz Corp

P O Box 374

Mendon, Utah 84325

http://www.jd-biz.com/

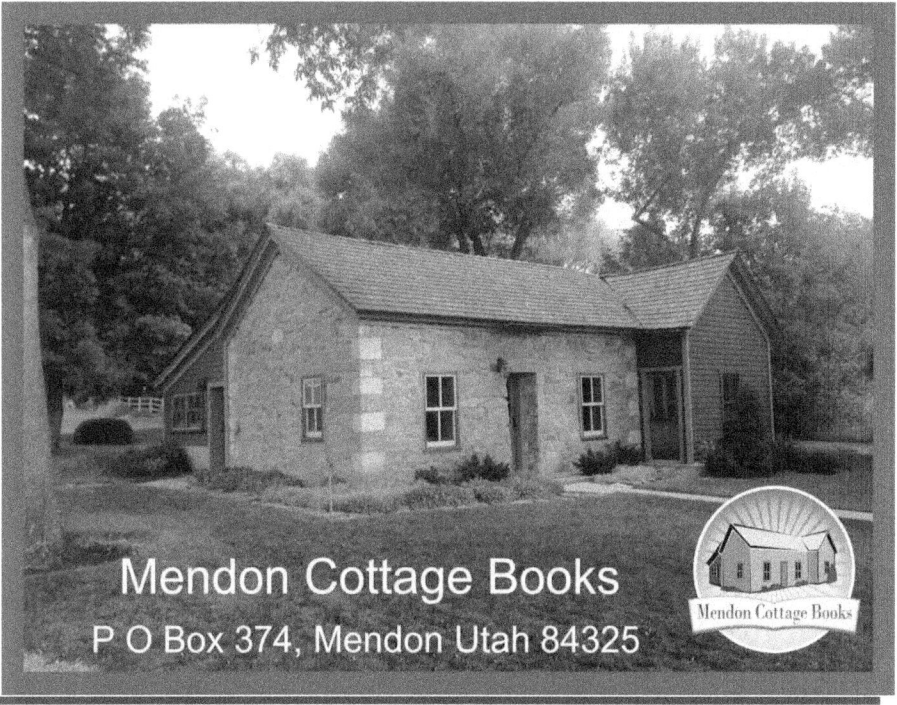